Umberto Sale

Encopresis – Poop on me

A case of encopresis resolved.

Book translated from Italian.

First edition: November 2014

Encopresis – Poop on me

A case of encopresis resolved

Umberto Sale

...to my children

Foreword

As I read about a therapy for encopresis online, shivers run down my spine, and I find myself thinking, "Thank goodness I didn't have to resort to all of this for my Marco." But perhaps Marco didn't need it? Maybe we resolved it differently with Marco because his case wasn't severe? And what if this same method could work for many other children?

I continue reading and share what I find, but the shivers persist:
"If the medical history and physical examination suggest a specific diagnosis of the disease, intestinal enemas should be performed to ensure regular bowel

movements. The initial treatment involves one to four cycles of the following regimen: on the first day, adult phosphate enemas (2 if the child is 7 years old); on the second day, a bisacodyl suppository (10 mg) rectally; on the third day, a bisacodyl capsule (5 mg) orally. To assess the effectiveness of the treatment, a follow-up abdominal X-ray is useful. Subsequent treatment (maintenance) involves administering multivitamin complexes (2/day) combined with light mineral oil, at doses of 15-30 ml orally twice a day for 4-6 months (or longer if daily bowel evacuation is necessary). Additional multivitamin complexes are needed because mineral oil interferes with vitamin absorption. (Note: Avoid mineral oil in infants and debilitated individuals due to the risk of inhalation.) A fiber-rich diet should be offered without forcing the child to ingest it. Additionally, at the appropriate time and for no more than 10 minutes, twice a day, the child should be seated on the toilet (preferably after meals). If necessary, after the initial treatment, oral laxatives may be administered in severe cases (e.g., senna, 5-10 ml/day) for 2-3 weeks, then every other day for 1 month. Relapses are common and, if identified early, should be treated with oral laxatives for 1-2 weeks. Mineral oil is gradually discontinued after 4-6 months of regular bowel emptying. If this regimen fails, further evaluations regarding diet and intestinal peristalsis are indicated."

With the information provided, I don't intend to question medical advice. Instead, I simply want to express my joy that I didn't subject my Marco to those treatments because I am now certain that he didn't need them and that he healed in a different way. We found another solution.

We resolved it!!

From the very first lines, I want to reassure the parents who are about to read this short book—parents who are desperate due to the significant little problem afflicting their little one, parents who, on various forums, have only found others with the same issue or have encountered learned doctors advising them to seek out specialists. But never has anyone said or recounted: "WE RESOLVED IT"; never has anyone announced: "We had the same encopresis problem with our son/daughter, AND WE RESOLVED IT." Well, dear parent friend, I announce to you that at the age of five and a half, we definitively and without relapse resolved our, rather our son Marco's, encopresis problem.

In this book, I aim to describe the journey undertaken by our family, composed of myself, Luca, the father, my wife Anna, our little Marco, and Marco's older sister, Mirella, who is three years his senior. I intend to narrate the doubts, methods, trials, experiments, illusions, and everything else my wife and I tried to overcome Marco's encopresis.

However, there are two premises I wish the reader to etch into their mind. Firstly, that I am solely a father, devoid of any medical or psychological knowledge, and thus this book is nothing more than a narrative where I expound upon my wholly personal theories borne from experience. It must be understood that these theories may lack any scientific foundation and could, perhaps, be erroneous. The second premise is that my deductions regarding the methodologies employed, which led to the resolution of my son Marco's encopresis, are entirely personal.

And at this very moment, as I refine the final corrections to the book you are reading on my computer, Marco, who will turn six in two months, calls out to me from the bathroom: "Daddy, come, I'm done pooping, come clean me up," and I burst with joy.

For my son Marco

Hello Marco,

Right now, you're just five and a half years old, and you've just learned how to read. I'm writing a story about your childhood experiences, but when you grow up, you might say to me, "Dad, you've turned one of my personal problems into a book, making it public domain. You're despicable!"

My dear son, I respond to you thus: what you deemed a problem was, in truth, a gift that distinguished you from birth and continues to do so today. A gift that, initially, your father failed to fully recognize: you were a child endowed with an extraordinary sensitivity, a sensitivity so deep that I find it difficult to express in words. It was a sensitivity you conveyed through the pure language of the heart, and which, my child, you taught me to understand and interpret. What we, in our ignorance, labeled as a problem, encopresis, was in fact merely a means of communication, a language reserved for children as remarkably sensitive as yourself, and understandable to adults only through the development of an equally profound emotional sensitivity.

What type of encopresis

Marco had always been a precocious child, learning early on to control his physiological need to urinate by quickly grasping the concept of using the toilet. Even at night, if he felt the urge, he would wake us to accompany him to the bathroom, and he hardly ever wet the bed. For this reason, we removed his diaper early, too early according to the pediatrician, and even too early in hindsight. We were completely unaware and had never even heard of encopresis. We simply thought he would eventually learn to defecate in the toilet and that he had constipation issues, so we tolerated his bowel movements in his underwear, indeed, we were pleased because the little stool released was a relief from his constipation. We were saddened by his constipation and worried about his apparent discomfort caused by constipation.

Then one day, I saw him standing, leaning against the door, straining to defecate, and I noticed something that sparked my first suspicion. He had his legs crossed while exerting himself to pass stool; crossing the legs at the knee was a posture more indicative of someone trying to hold back stool than of a child trying to push it out. If he wanted to help himself pass stool, he would have spread his legs rather than crossing them. I decided to observe him more closely, and I realized I was right. He wasn't constipated, and even if he was, he wasn't aiding the defecation process; instead, he was holding it in and letting it out very slowly, using this strange practice of crossing his legs. From that day on, around Marco's age of three and a half, our torment began, and when I say "our," I mean Marco's as well. He started to understand that I was watching him while he withheld his stool, disregarding our initial patient suggestions to sit on the toilet, and began to hide and remove himself from our sight during his act of withholding stool.

Thus began our sad days, lasting for over a year.

Pediatrician luminary

...and so my wife and I sought out the best pediatrician in the city, and we found a luminary, a renowned university professor.

In the esteemed pediatrician's office, the examination of my son lasted almost an hour, and to be honest, I was also disheartened by the professor's persistence in searching for any cognitive issues in my little Marco. The search ended with the professor's surrender, who declared that in his opinion, my Marco was a child even more intelligent than his average of observed children and without any growth disorders. He advised us to perform a slightly more invasive examination for our son to check for any intestinal or rectal problems. My wife and I never had Marco undergo those exams to avoid distressing him, and thankfully, I can say we never did. Then, the "luminary" also recommended a conditioning therapy, that is, to have Marco sit on the toilet at regular intervals for a certain number of minutes to instill a proper habit in him. And when we returned home, the tough struggle and attempts at conditioning began.

Marco absolutely refused to even consider sitting; he squirmed, cried, screamed. It seemed as if when we made him sit on the toilet, we were pulling out his fingernails. His was an invincible terror of the toilet, and after a few weeks of screams, problems, attempts with kindness, with severity, with promises, with our feigned tears because he wouldn't sit, and with the most imaginative attempts concocted by us parents, we surrendered to Marco. Our conditioning attempts suggested by the pediatrician all failed, one after the other.

The pediatrician also advised us to enroll Marco in preschool. This was to facilitate his separation from his mother. Indeed, Marco and his mother were morbidly and physically always attached to each other; it seemed as if the umbilical cord had never been severed. So, we enrolled Marco in preschool. He took to preschool with philosophy and without much regret, and at preschool, he never soiled his underwear; he saved it for home.

The toilet gnome

"You know, Marco, there's a tiny gnome, ever so kind, who brings a little gift to children when they sit on the toilet."

"This is a little story and a suggestion I read on the internet after browsing through dozens of forums frequented by desperate moms dealing with their little ones' encopresis. And so I bled out, dozens of gifts brought by the gnome!! Yes, the method worked for the conditioning dictated by the pediatrician; Marco would sit on the toilet, but far from dawning on him that he had to sit there to defecate, he sat only for the little gift. The bathroom was just a cunning tool to get the gift, after which he would retreat to a corner, cross-legged, to defecate. So, screw the toilet gnome! Perhaps some parents will tell me they've had a positive effect from the toilet gnome, but it wasn't the case for us, and if I ever come across this damn consumerist gnome, I swear I'll kill it!!"

Brother Psychologist

I have a brother who is a psychologist. As you well know, psychologists cannot psychoanalyze their relatives, and not only did my brother not want to do it, but he also tried not to confront my wife's resistance to seeing a psychologist; it was actually my wife who didn't believe in psychology, a bit of distrust towards this science is quite common, especially in those who have never seen a psychologist, and I understood, and perhaps even shared, my wife's distrust, but I was desperate and would have tried any form of witchcraft just to solve the problem of encopresis. But then I realized that many people, myself included, interpret psychologists in the same way the Inquisition tribunal interpreted the theory of heliocentrism. Dear parents, my brother Duilio instead guided us towards the slow but sudden solution to Marco's encopresis problem. Thanks to him and psychologist Alessandra, we understood why my wife and I were suffering from encopresis, yes, you read that right, I was the problem, not Marco. This last one is a personal consideration that I will detail in the rest of the writing. Returning to my brother, he simply asked me how we slept and in which rooms and beds, my wife, my daughter Mirella, Marco, and I. I replied that we all slept in the master bedroom and I slept on the outermost side of the bed, next to me slept my daughter, then next to my daughter slept my wife, and then at the other end of the double bed, next to my wife slept Marco. In practice, Marco and I were at the outermost side of the bed, and my daughter was between my wife and me. My brother simply suggested that I shouldn't let my daughter Mirella sleep between my wife and me, but instead let Marco sleep in the middle. At first, I hadn't even noticed that it was my daughter sleeping between us parents and not Marco, and I accepted the suggestion, but I never would have thought that simple suggestion would be the turning point, that suggestion was the secret code to open the door to my son Marco's problem. Thanks to my brother Duilio, without realizing it, I had started a year earlier on the path to solving encopresis, or rather, I will say, to understanding the encopretic language spoken by Marco.

Tragic nature of encopresis

As Marco grew, his feces became more adult-like, larger and smellier. Imagine always having the stench of feces in your nose. Guests come over, and you feel uncomfortable because of the smell! You go to friends' houses, and the smell follows you! You hug your son, and the smell triples! You constantly clean feces from his underwear, or out of desperation, the underwear becomes disposable, throwing away one or more soiled ones every day. You have to cover the sofas and armchairs to prevent them from permanently smelling like feces. You find small pieces of feces around the house that have escaped from your son's pants, and even worse, your friends find the fecal bits on the floor of their home because they've leaked from your son's pant legs.

You're afraid to go to restaurants, afraid to be invited to dinner; you're forced to explain your son's problem to alleviate the embarrassment of the constant stench that accompanies the whole family.

When he poops

Marco is a lover of live or fake animals; he has dozens of plastic ones and only plays with them. He lines them up, sorts them by species, divides them into herbivores, carnivores, and omnivores. He spends hours playing with the animals and relaxes a lot doing so. It's while he's playing with the animals that he defecates in his underwear, with an attitude that mixes effort in holding it in and pleasure in releasing it slowly. In doing so, he reminded me of the attitude I might have while smoking a good Tuscan cigar and sipping on a good rum, simultaneously engaged in something that requires a small physical effort. Other times, the urge to defecate was sudden, so he would run far away from my sight, and I would see him standing, leaning against a door or a couch, with crossed legs and a red face from the effort of holding back the violence of the feces trying to escape. In practice, two methodologies, if you'll allow me to use the term: the first, in relaxation mode with a slow and prolonged release of feces, even under our eyes; the second, sudden and violent feces retention, away from our eyes and perhaps due to a stronger and more sudden physiological stimulus.

The Psychologist

Until Marco was four years and six months old, my wife and I, self-taught with methods picked up here and there, tried in every way to solve the problem of encopresis. We tried gentle methods, slightly tougher ones, promises, threats—believe me, we tried everything. Then finally, I asked my brother to recommend a psychologist, even if I had to go alone if my wife opposed it. My brother suggested his psychologist friend, who, in his opinion, was very good and would offer us a discounted rate due to her friendship with him. When you mention a psychologist around here, people often associate the profession with those who have severe mental imbalances and are forced to see a doctor. This couldn't be more wrong. Over these few months, I've come to understand how much a psychologist can improve your quality of life, even if you think you have no problems. A good, intelligent, and well-prepared psychologist can enhance your quality of life. If I had the financial means, I would go to a psychologist every week, like going to a gym or engaging in a sport, not for the body but for the mind. From Marco's age of four and a half, for about eight months, we visited Dr. Alessandra twice a week. Already after the first day, we felt stronger, with a powerful ally by our side. Before starting the visits with the psychologist, I thought I had a strong sensitivity in considering my son and my relationship with him. Instead, Dr. Alessandra made me realize, without ever saying it directly, that I was like an elephant walking among the ceramics of my son's mental sensitivity. She made me understand the importance of firmness, the inconsistency and sterility of anger, the importance of the relationship, and the awareness of the mask that can exist in a relationship, a mask that sometimes hides what is not a real bond with your child. Over time, the elephant walking among the ceramics of my son's sensitivities was transforming into a feather that caressed and understood them. Marco started making his first "poops" in the toilet. His first serious attempt was after returning home from Dr. Alessandra's office, and the first real time happened while he was taking a warm bath in the tub. He was alone in the bathroom with his little animal toys, bathing in the tub. He got up from the tub without us noticing and called out to us, or rather, he called me: "Dad, daddy, come see something beautiful." We found him on the toilet, defecating, and it was true, perhaps it was the first time I saw a bit of my son's feces in the toilet. For many months, Dr. Alessandra worked on my wife and me, and perhaps less on my son. I appreciated the significant work she did on me; maybe she did a lot of work on my wife too, but I think each person perceives and expresses more the work developed on themselves. So much so that today, I think I was the cause of my son's soiling in his underwear. Maybe my wife thinks the same about herself, but I'm the one writing this book, so I'm telling you about my experience. You know, Dr. Alessandra's technique is very particular. I don't know if it's hers or all psychologists', but she doesn't tell you anything at all. You expect a psychologist to tell you something like: "Your child has this problem because you adopt this or that wrong behavior." But it's not like that. The psychologist makes sure that you yourself can find the answer and understand what your wrong behaviors are. The consistency of visits to the psychologist is useful so that there are no relapses. Dr. Alessandra first made me understand my presumption of perfection in my relationship with my son. I thought I was giving my all to my son, but it wasn't true. She suggested I dedicate more time to him, brought to my awareness that I wasn't dedicating the right amount of time to my son, and if I did, maybe I did it more out of obligation. She probably knew that this obligation would have to transform into pleasure to solve my son's problem, but initially, she suggested it as a duty, trusting in its future transformation into pleasure. In fact, I adored and still adore my first daughter Mirella; I felt she was mine, a part of me, a feeling perhaps driven also by my physical resemblance to her. Often, my relationship with my son was dictated solely by the fairness of treatment compared to my first daughter, and perhaps not by genuine desire. It was right that I divided my time and myself with Marco and Mirella for reasons of fairness. It was right and fair that my son Marco also slept in the middle between me and my wife, and so he began to sleep between us two for reasons of fairness. Fairness was the problem of encopresis! The feces held back by my son, his unhealthy attachment to his mother, was a deficiency in my relationship with Marco, a realization in Marco of his extreme sensitivity, that I was with him only for fairness. Let me be clear: mine was a latent deficiency in the relationship, one no parent would have noticed without the intervention of a psychologist educating your mind and making you understand how much infinite and great sensitivity a 4-year-old child can have more than us, and how many of your feelings, even the most hidden from yourself, your child can grasp. I saw a world of feelings and relationships with my son in black and white; he saw a world of sensitivity in colors and high definition. I was my son's feces!! I was the feces my son wanted to keep with him. Until I became a part of Marco like his feces, my son would never let go of his feces in the toilet.

Small relapse

It's been two months now since Marco only uses the toilet to defecate. My house smells delightful, the bathroom is spotless, Marco's underwear is washed with the rest of the family's laundry—in short, a newfound and renewed serenity every day.

Summer vacation is almost here, and my motorcycle insurance is due, as is my car insurance. Only those who live in the province of Naples, despite being in the top insurance class for years, know what it means to pay an unjustifiably expensive insurance premium for any means of transportation.

Then, on top of insurance, there are a couple of unexpected home repair expenses, and finally, the cost of the vacation. I become acutely aware that after more than twenty years of work, my salary is very low compared to many other jobs. A slight form of depression creeps in, accompanied by anger for the job that, despite the sleepless nights and overtime, yields me nothing more. Unbeknownst to me, the sensitivity indicator in my son Marco reignites, and he starts soiling his underwear again.

I talk to him about it, I hug him, I embrace him with all the love I have, but the sensitivity indicator in his brain is infallible, of an otherworldly precision and reliability. My son senses me withdrawing, and he holds back his feces once again, which, strangely enough, represents me. In a much lighter form, much lighter than before, he falls back into the problem. Indeed, he says he's soiled his underwear a bit and goes to do the "big one" in the toilet. But even my form of distancing from Marco is slight, yet detected by the extremely sensitive sensor placed in the sensitivity of little Marco.

The Sister

Marco has an older sister, Mirella, who is three years his senior. Mirella is an incredibly calm, obedient, lively, and intelligent girl. It's only fair that I speak of her, both to make the family picture more understandable and because, in the end, she deserves some glory for having endured, poor little thing, the negative consequences of Marco's encopresis.

She, too, has tried every avenue to help Marco, acting as a driving force for the parents in the excitement of our anti-encopresis techniques. Mirella has always been committed to implementing our practices. She didn't rebel against my distancing from her and the corresponding closeness to Marco, but she surely must have suffered from it. Unfortunately, a parent must always intervene with the weaker child, even at the cost of arousing jealousy and misunderstandings. Therefore, I am grateful to Mirella as well, who with her understanding and tolerance, took my distancing well and understood the importance of my behavior as a mature child.

The relationship between Marco and Mirella has always been excellent. They argue very little, and Marco, in particular, adores his sister. He sees her as a role model and treasures all her teachings. Mirella also has an excellent relationship with me; we are connected in an inexplicable way, and Marco has understood this well, even before the bond between me and Marco became of the same kind.

Dividing a parent's love between two children is as difficult as balancing a stationary bicycle. But I have learned to balance the bike, and Marco has recovered.

Sensibility

And now, the epilogue: how to heal from encopresis. I already know that I will rewrite this chapter many times in an attempt to express in words the cure for encopresis, a cure in which the patient, contrary to what one might suppose, is the father in my case. In fact, as I have already told you before, the real patient with problems was me, and therefore my son was only trying to make me understand through his very personal "encopretic language" my pathology.

I have spoken to you about the awareness gained thanks to psychologist Alessandra that I was not dedicating enough time to my son and the awareness gained thanks to my brother, a psychologist, that Marco did not sleep between us parents but closer to the mother, as it was Mirella who slept between the father and the mother.

Over time, these incorrect behaviors of mine have been corrected with diligent and systematic fulfillment of my duties and time distribution. But day after day, dedicating more time to Marco, sleeping next to him, getting closer and more connected, was transforming, was perfecting. In the evening, upon returning from my work, the fulfillment of the schematic duty was gradually changing, becoming pleasure, desire, eagerness. The bond was becoming tighter, the love, the pleasure of total contact, the desire to be close to Marco was taking over, even to the point where I felt withdrawal symptoms from being away from Marco. And when this passion of mine became irresistible, impossible to explain due to its immensity, when this passion broke the chains that kept Marco eagerly tied to his mother, when this passion became total, constant, solely driven by my perpetual desire, surpassing the times suggested by the psychologist, when my love and connection became total, physical, mental, and irresistible, my son was healed! Only then did my son throw away his poop in the toilet. He didn't need it anymore! Because now he had me, completely, with all my strength, with all my love, and he immediately sensed it.

I, as a father, took the place of his poop! His poop was me, and his real poop went to hell in the toilet! It was me who now warmed him, not his poop. It was me who shared his moments of tranquility while playing with his plastic animals, not his poop. It was me attached to his little body at night, not his poop. I was his poop. And now, at the mere thought of encopresis, I am overwhelmed with the urge to run to him, hold him close, kiss him, and embrace him with all the love and passion in the world, and then some. *"Hello dear mothers and fathers, it's Marco speaking, just five and a half years old, and I want to explain to you in the words of grown-ups what the poop in my underwear is: it's an incredibly advanced form of language that you adults find difficult to understand. It's a language where you don't need your brain to understand, where you don't need your ears to listen, and where you don't need your eyes to see. It's a language where only by opening your heart to us little ones will you gradually learn to understand, and the more your heart opens, the better we'll be able to communicate with you grown-ups."*

Gift

"Dad, I've explained it to you so many times, but maybe you're missing a little gear in your brain? I've told you that you give me a gift, and I give you a gift." "What gift, Marco?" "That thing, Daddy, the poop!" "And what gift do I have to give you, Marco?" To this question, I would have expected a response like a toy, an animal, but instead little Marco says, "When you come home from work, we play soccer one time, volleyball another time, and go biking together another time."

This dialogue occurred after a small setback in Marco's encopresis following two consecutive months of completely defeating the problem with Marco's underwear immaculate and "big poops" in the toilet. Now it has resurfaced but in a milder form where we can communicate with Marco, and where, if caught at the onset of the urge, he goes to poop in the toilet, only minimally soiling his underwear. And now that I'm handling my work-related financial issues better, Marco is gradually returning to normalcy. There's almost a one-to-one relationship between the concept of the gift and the poop. Where the gift for my son is a game with dad, be it soccer or volleyball, but perhaps for your little one it could be a bike ride or a kiss between mom and dad. It's up to you to learn to read your child's intricate language.

Chocolate and chili pepper

Chocolate has never been a delicacy for Marco, but that's not what I want to talk to you about. Chocolate represents the reward, the praise, the embrace for Marco's first "poopies" in the toilet; the chili pepper represents the threat of sending him to boarding school.

Marco's sister always knew what I meant by boarding school, and she carefully explained to her little brother that boarding school was the place where naughty children go and those who poop their pants to make them learn to do it in the toilet, where there are adults who don't hesitate to hit children, and where you don't sleep with your parents at night - quite a terrifying discussion for a five-year-old. Indeed, Marco was terrified at the thought of us sending him to boarding school.

After his recovery, I deeply regretted scaring Marco about boarding school, but that doesn't change the fact that, in addition to the complete rebuilding of our father-son relationship, the fear of boarding school also contributed about 10 or 20 percent. In fact, during the relapse period, when our relationship with Marco was one of established love but perhaps not renewed due to work-related issues, I brought up the threat of boarding school again.

But Marco insists on the concept of the gift. This wonderful gift represented by my time that he wants his daddy to dedicate to him, in exchange for his poop in the toilet.

This is the key to everything; encopresis is just a form of non-verbal communication from the child that highlights and attempts to communicate some behavioral and emotional shortcomings in our relationship with him. I wanted to talk to you about boarding school only for the sake of completeness, but I beg you, dear parents, to understand that the key to solving your problem is not punishment but loving communication.

Reward Them

Empower your encopretic little ones, make them proud of their abilities, call them champions, never humiliate them. As soon as a good opportunity arises, tell them, "Dad is proud of you," "You're my champion!"

Holidays

Away from the thoughts of my work, away from the computer, I discover Marco's great aptitude for swimming. We play together in the pool, he trusts me implicitly and without fear he dives into the deep water, confident that his dad won't let him drown. Our physical contact increases as he begins to play-fight with me, where for me, the play-fight is nothing more than an opportunity for physical contact and embrace with my son. He literally steals my attention away from my daughter, directing it towards him.

The vacation home in the resort is small

and we're practically always together. He can't hide to poop and tries not to do it at all, but then the natural urge becomes irresistible and he goes to poop in the toilet.

The vacation was one of the first signs of how powerful the bond between Marco and me was, leading him to make his first poops or attempts in the toilet. Of course, if I had spent the vacation fishing and playing soccer, I wouldn't have had this positive response from Marco. This is to tell you how important attention is in the therapy of encopresis, attention that must not be repressive or controlling, but only affectionate. In the small environment of the vacation village cottage, the attention was focused on Marco, and being only affectionate attention, it achieved its result. When I saw that Marco wanted to poop but held back, I would jokingly make him sit on the toilet and hug him tightly, and even if he didn't poop, I understood that he sensed I was learning to translate his deep "encopretic language."

Children

Children who speak late, children who stutter, encopretic children…how many languages do our little ones speak, how much sensitivity is expressed in those reactions? We tend to provide a rational explanation, dictated by intellect and our culture, but we don't hear, we don't understand.

Only if we revolutionize and adapt our cognitive form can we understand that it is the Earth that revolves around the sun, despite believing the opposite for thousands of years. It's tough for an adult to acknowledge that despite your studies, your life experience, your intellect, a five-year-old speaks an extremely advanced language that you may only partially understand.

Year 2024

I asked my 15-year-old son, with whom I have a wonderful relationship, why he used to hold in his bowel movements as a child; not so easily, he replied that it was a form of pleasure, but that when he decided to go to the bathroom, the accumulated feces were too much and required too much effort to expel.

My son has solved the problem for years; he is a balanced, intelligent, sociable young man…the son everyone would want to have.

Summary

- Foreword 4
- We resolved it!! 7
- For my son Marco 11
- What type of encopresis 13
- Pediatrician luminary 16
- The toilet gnome 19
- Brother Psychologist 21
- Tragic nature of encopresis 24
- When he poops 26
- The Psychologist 28
- Small relapse 35
- The Sister 38
- Sensibility 41
- Gift 45
- Chocolate and chili pepper 47
- Reward Them 50
- Holidays 51
- Children 54
  - Year 2024 56
- Summary 57

www.ingramcontent.com/pod-product-compliance
Lightning Source LLC
Chambersburg PA
CBHW050243230526
45470CB00005B/2092